Table of Contents

Blood Tests for Exocrine Pancreatic Insufficiency (EPI): Understanding the Diagnostic Process

1. Introduction to Exocrine Pancreatic Insufficiency (EPI)

2. Importance of Accurate Diagnosis

3. Clinical Symptoms and Signs of EPI

4. Role of Blood Tests in Diagnosing EPI

4.1. 1.1 Pancreatic Enzyme Levels in Blood

4.2. 1.2 Other Blood Markers for EPI Diagnosis

5. Comparison with Other Diagnostic Methods

6. Interpreting Blood Test Results

7. Challenges and Limitations of Blood Tests for EPI Diagnosis

8. Future Directions in EPI Diagnosis Research

9. Conclusion and Summary

Understanding Exocrine Pancreatic Insufficiency (EPI): Diagnosis and Management

1. Introduction to Exocrine Pancreatic Insufficiency (EPI)

2. Signs and Symptoms of EPI

3. Diagnostic Approaches for EPI

3.1. Blood Tests for EPI

3.2. Stool Tests for EPI

4. Differential Diagnosis of EPI

5. Management of EPI

5.1. Enzyme Replacement Therapy

5.2. Nutritional Support

6. Complications Associated with Untreated EPI

7. Prognosis and Quality of Life in EPI

8. Research and Future Directions in EPI

Blood Tests for Exocrine Pancreatic Insufficiency (EPI): Understanding the Diagnostic Process

1. Introduction to Exocrine Pancreatic Insufficiency (EPI)

However, before reaching a firm diagnosis, the vet will need to rule out other causes of the symptoms and consider likely probabilities. It can (for the most part) be definitively diagnosed and managed with a simple diet and enzyme supplementation. This means that accurate testing is of high priority because incorrect diagnosis could result in multiple other diagnostic procedures, unnecessary treatments, and a reduced quality of life for the animal. One way we work up a diagnosis of EPI is to use blood tests assessing the levels of various blood proteins in dogs and cats. These help with the diagnosis, especially if those blood tests are abnormal. In those cases, the dog may well have EPI.

Exocrine pancreatic insufficiency (EPI) occurs when the pancreas can't produce enough enzymes to break down food. Food isn't absorbed properly in the small intestine and instead passes into the large intestine where it is broken down by bacteria, which can cause some very unpleasant symptoms. EPI can occur in dogs and cats, as well as having a range of underlying causes such as pancreatitis, a dietary intolerance, or pancreatic acinar atrophy (where the cells in the pancreas that produce the enzymes are slowly destroyed). It can happen at any age and in any breed. Once diagnosed, management usually involves supplementation with pancreatic enzymes that are added to food.

2. Importance of Accurate Diagnosis

There are several tests used to diagnose EPI in human beings. Before you choose a single test to describe, it may be worth considering presenting the various tests in a more general compartments - indirect tests (such as faecal elastase) that show lack of pancreatic function, direct pancreatic function tests such as the secretin/cholecystokinin test. The Elastase-1 stool test is the preferred test in humans with EPI. There are also blood tests that aid in the diagnosis of EPI; these are used with the faecal blood tests. Using a combination of these tests can increase the specificity of the diagnosis of EPI. In human medicine, the use of combinations of these blood tests has the same sensitivity and specificity as the stool test for faecal elastase. We tend to use the serum TLI measurements as this tests the functionality of the remaining tissue as EPI patients can still have hyperplasia of the exocrine gland giving rise to a large serum protein measurement depending on what test is used.

The aim of this section is to impress upon the reader the importance of getting a definitive diagnosis for EPI. This is important because accurate diagnosis is the basis for managing a condition effectively and tailoring appropriate treatment for that condition. This provides logic for the next section of the manuscript. There are a number of clinical indications of EPI in human medicine but no data currently available on whether the signs we are using to diagnose EPI can be somebody anything else. There are some signs that are termed non-specific but are typically seen in these patients, therefore contributing to the overall clinical picture. It would make sense to include some text about non-specific signs that also contribute to the diagnosis of EPI in the section. Other signs and symptoms of EPI may be included (this is not an exhaustive list - please refer to original documents when writing the manuscript).

3. Clinical Symptoms and Signs of EPI

Exocrine pancreatic insufficiency or EPI is a decreased capability of the pancreas to produce digestive enzymes that help the body convert food into usable nutrients. Pancreatic enzymes include amylase to digest carbohydrates, lipase to digest fats into fatty acids, and trypsin and other proteases to digest proteins into amino acids. These digestive enzymes are secreted in an active form; to avoid auto-digestion (pancreatitis), zymogens (inactivated enzymes) are replaced with proenzymes as appropriate, for example, trypsinogen is activated by enterokinase and converted into trypsin. EPI generally develops when at least 85-90% of the pancreas is no longer viable; at which point both enzyme and hormone (insulin) production from the pancreas are severely impaired. The most common causes of EPI in dogs are chronic pancreatitis, pancreatic acinar atrophy (PAA), neoplasia (carcinoma), exocrine pancreatic insufficiency, and severe fibrosis. In cats, chronic pancreatitis is the main cause of pancreatic exocrine insufficiency.

Clients with EPI can present with weight loss (76-91%), loose/fatty stool (steatorrhea; 63-74%), and diarrhea (22-72%). Many clients with EPI also show signs of malnutrition with decreased serum concentrations of albumin (34-59%) and folate (25-50%) and anemia (9-12%). Vitamin and mineral co-morbidities including hypocalcemia, hypomagnesemia, hypokalemia, hypophosphatemia, and hypocholesterolemia may also be seen. Gastrointestinal symptoms such as gas and abdominal pain are less specific for EPI, present only in approximately 25% of cases, and are more consistent with symptoms of small intestinal dysbiosis. The lack of clinical specificity in the presenting clinical symptoms and signs indicates that further diagnostic testing is needed to facilitate a definitive diagnosis of EPI.

4. Role of Blood Tests in Diagnosing EPI

Blood test detection of EPI is essential in diagnostic efforts, as EPI is essentially related to an imbalance of nutrients in one's bloodstream. Consequently, some of the established indicators for blood testing include several blood markers, along with acinar enzyme candidates. In practice, carbohydrate and fat malabsorption demonstrably relate to low elastase 1 levels and weight loss to document the clinical impact of low elastase 1 or fecal fat levels, and both tests correlate well with each other. Non-invasive blood tests for EPI typically rely on measuring the activity or level of the candidate enzyme from the pancreas which is exhausted first in the disease course. These are typically trypsin and chymotrypsin activity in the serum or pancreolauryl levels in the urine. This article relies on a more biochemical approach to blood tests. It should be noted that some liver disorders may mimic EPI serum, like alpha-1-antitrypsin deficiency, adenohypophyseal hormone deficiency, chronic hemodialysis, chronic pancreatitis, cystic fibrosis, fibrocystic disease of the pancreas, idiopathic steatorrhea, and primary biliary liver cirrhosis.

Distinguishing a healthy pancreas from one affected by EPI requires significant investigative effort. Besides evidence-based medical history and symptoms, the focus is mostly on non-invasive imaging or blood tests, yet other means for early recognition of EPI remain largely experimented, including genetic testing. It stands to reason that a great deal of scientific research has been invested into investigating blood tests, mainly due to their ease of administration and ability to determine various effector molecules which would confirm or deny the case for EPI.

4.1. 1.1 Pancreatic Enzyme Levels in Blood

Some of the fat digestion products are useful for diagnosing EPI, often as an additional tool in individuals with unexplained gastrointestinal symptoms. Blood contains a range of different substances and some studies have assessed if certain enzymes produced by the pancreas, or their byproducts, can be found in blood and may be useful for diagnosing EPI. Blood markers are used to see if an individual might have EPI and require further investigation, for example, a special test called a faecal elastase test or a secretin stimulation test, which are the best ways to diagnose EPI. If you are diagnosed with EPI, these blood tests can also be used annually to monitor changes in the progression of the disease over time.

A widely available, quick and non-invasive way to measure the levels of pancreatic enzymes is by blood tests. These tests primarily assess for the presence of the digestive enzymes amylase and lipase. There are no internationally agreed levels, or cut-offs, above which these enzymes can be said to be abnormal. Constructs - standard ranges - differ among laboratories and across countries due to differences in measurement techniques, reagents, operator variability, and the reference populations used in calculations. This means the results of tests for amylase and lipase must be compared with the laboratory constructs. However, lipase can be more informative than amylase. Amylase may be reabsorbed in the kidney, giving rise to a low profile, while lipase is excreted via the colon, maintaining a flat profile.

4.2. 1.2 Other Blood Markers for EPI Diagnosis

In this context, another marker may also be found in blood, the fecal elastase-1 concentration, protein detected in the stool or blood, the measurements of which can be used to detect EPI. Elastase-1 is a major component of the pancreas and is characterized as an excretory digestive enzyme. The evaluation of elastase-1 is effective and simple for outpatient diagnosis of pancreatic exocrine insufficiency (EPI). Moreover, with the negative endoscopy results, the decrease not only in the concentration of elastase-1 but also in the concentration of elastase-1 in the bloodstream can be a guide to suspect the presence of subclinical EPI. Fecal elastase-1 was mildly decreased. Plum and serum elastase-1 have been used many times to guide patients to diagnose exocrine pancreatic insufficiency (EPI) and as a marker for EPI. Serum elastase-1.

This section will provide reasons why drawing blood for EPI diagnosis is efficient in clinical settings and how elastase-1 compares to other severe markers when using blood for diagnosis. One of the possible markers in the blood for EPI diagnosis is the cobalamin concentration in the blood. However, as mentioned earlier, the concentration of cobalamin is still subject to variations and can even remain normal in some patients with EPI. Normally, the cobalamin concentration is lower in the blood of EPI patients. Even if a low cobalamin concentration in the blood could indirectly suggest EPI, cobalamin is not directly recommended for the diagnosis of

EPI. Overall, taking into account the patient's clinical condition, it is not ideal to rely only on the cobalamin concentration in blood when diagnosing EPI.

5. Comparison with Other Diagnostic Methods

Indeed, blood tests may provide the same level of accuracy – among other things, accuracy should be higher than that of the 72% correct answers through clinical symptoms only – without the need for strict sample preparation and with greater retrospective flexibility. The faecal test's limitation is the necessity to suspend for some days large doses of enzymes before collection, which some patients reported led them to feel better possible symptoms despite never having presented any symptoms (#25), which would make them reluctant to conducting the test. However, blood tests present some inherent observer-dependent variability, and the results appear to be limited by the lack of a consensual upper reference standard for the 13C-Ubt. However, with an explicitly developed interpretation strategy such as what we presented in this study, the impact of those limitations is minimized.

Comparing with other diagnostic methods: Although there are two other tests that are available for the diagnosis of exocrine pancreatic insufficiency (EPI) simultaneously – faecal elastase and the 13C-labeled mixed triglycerides breath test (which is available in only a small number of laboratories so far), a blood test would offer a rapid and direct alternative. Furthermore, when possible, at conferences and in guideline groups, attending physicians expressed the preference of their (asymptomatic) patients for a blood test over faecal tests.

6. Interpreting Blood Test Results

- It is desirable to carry out tests in a state of fasting and in the morning when the pancreatic function is in a state of high activity. - An excess volume of enzymes and inhibitors can be eliminated by alternately performing various methods of evaluation using blood and stool. - When assessing the cause of exocrine insufficiency, it is advisable to study the functional state of the stomach to exclude concomitant pathology of the gastroduodenal region. In this case, the research of the secretory function of the stomach in the basal period and after stimulation is performed. - In the presence of acute symptoms of exocrine insufficiency of the pancreas, it is advisable to evaluate the current level of spirituality and anxiety. At the same time, it is noted that the achieved level of spirituality and anxiety correlates with the severity of exocrine pancreatic insufficiency. Given that APS is significantly more relevant for women, the level of anxiety and spirituality is higher in women with APS than in men.

When assessing a patient with possible EPI, the interpretation of blood test results is crucial for diagnosing the disease. For these purposes, GPs have three blood sample methods such as laboratory PANCREOLAURINS, IMMUNOLOGICAL TEST, P-Amylase blood tests. When interpreting blood test results, there are the following rules:

Recently, respected researchers and companies have discussed the latest achievements and findings in pancreatic exocrine insufficiency at the ASPIRE conference in Barcelona. In the next few weeks, we will discuss a few of the key aspects of the diagnosis and management of EPI that were covered.

7. Challenges and Limitations of Blood Tests for EPI Diagnosis

In conclusion, suggesting that the commercial pancreas-specific lipase is not sufficient for the diagnosis of EPI. Future research should focus on trying to identify not only the most selective and optimal pancreas-specific lipase content but also one that may differentiate between RSPL of pancreatic as opposed to the non-pancreatic ROI.

The place of RSPL serum measurements in addition to other pancreas-specific lipase formulations remains to be elucidated.

Before implementation of pancreas-specific lipase tests into clinical practice, clinical performance of pancreas-specific lipase tests should be more convincingly studied, preferably head-to-head in the same clinical cohorts.

In conclusion, evidence suggests that 4 different pancreas-specific lipase serum tests should be evaluated in additional clinical performance studies to further understand their potential in diagnostics. Additional studies on pancreas-specific lipase are required, but testing directly on duodenal fluid might provide an alternative with more clinical potential for the future.

Currently, several drawbacks elaborated further prevent the implementation of pancreas-specific lipase blood tests into regular clinical practice for EPI diagnosis to be able to compete with other direct and surrogate EPI tests.

Identifying diagnostic tools for EPI is a complex process. Several challenges exist, which may impede the further development and propagation of blood tests for pancreas-specific lipase in regular clinical practice.

8. Future Directions in EPI Diagnosis Research

In conclusion, we believe that there is a need for future direction in both diagnostic capability and drug development, with perhaps improvements in the sensors, passing or exploiting the sub-clinical phase of EPI, or reaching patients with earlier therapy obtained through drug development. In order to develop appropriate diagnostic markers, it is possible that currently available techniques could be used to discover whether measurement of enzyme and fat should be combined into one test or taken individually for the best results. Further, enrollment of appropriate control group samples such as those sensitive to EPI may facilitate de novo discovery of plasma/urine EPI diagnostic tests.

Future directions in EPI diagnosis research will focus on discovering novel biomarkers and drug development to inform and expand on current therapies. Given the investment in CF, and the other commonest disease associated with EPI, diabetes; drug development could feasibly be expedited from compounds being developed for these conditions to EPI. However, given the rapidly advancing non-surgical treatments for diabetes, and the fact that glucose intolerance in non-surgical pancreatic cancer, at least soon diminishes drastically if not improves, it seems unlikely that EPI-specific therapy could help many adult patients with CP and PDAC. Moreover, glucose intolerance, whilst it remains mild or diet-controlled, is less of an issue with regard to weight and may not see nutritional status deteriorate significantly. Long term, research into the ability of sustained therapy with pancreatin to slow or prevent the onset of diabetes in CP and PDAC will be considered.

One of the major criticisms of the published observational/cohort studies was the lack of sensitivity; notably false negatives. Taking an ethical standpoint, researchers need to be certain that sufficient innovative thought has gone into the control group selection to ensure maximum patient safety, and without such levels of certainty, findings are unlikely to get any funding. Indeed, many funded studies have had to rethink the patient population and are therefore starting from an observation point (to determine ideally where the cut-points are for 'normal' subjects using healthy volunteers or those with mild disease rather than how any test performs). It remains to be seen, however, whether novel biomarker and/or metabolomic tests, which are less dependent on an intact pancreas (enzymes and bicarbonate), but instead are markers of underlying exocrine pancreatic function in humans, will be seen to be cost-effective measures in EPI.

9. Conclusion and Summary

Technical challenges are the vague gold standard, potential inherent limitations (e.g. body size limit, intolerance, inhalation nervousness to the patient, risks due to radiation), or the challenges for workup of adverse events (e.g. radiation dose exposure, oversight, time consumption, ICU transportation, need for follow up of the patient) associated with the invasive assessments. On the other hand, non-PET investigations are unhelpful in many patients with EPI, cannot accurately record light EPI, are impractical and/or difficult for ICU patients, have not been widespread in broad practice, and are very restricted, particularly during a pandemic, with inoperative GI manometry centers. It should be emphasized that it is equally important that the new test could not only be less invasive and simple but would help a clinician and an intensivist to optimize the ratio of pancreatic insufficiency/type and dose of any enzyme preparation administered to their patients. However, no novel such blood EPI or other GI insufficiency test has been suggested thus far. Hence, in conclusion, the suggested potential future research directions in GI enzyme insufficiency are numerous from their exact position in the clinical assessment of ICU problems. The definitive universal EPI test would be simple, atraumatic, fast-acting, accurate, informative, affordable, safe, and non-invasive. Although a variety of wild options might work well enough, no such EPI or GI function test is yet available in capabilities.

EPI is associated with malnutrition because of malabsorption, which can only develop if >90% of pancreatic acinar tissue is destroyed. It is clinically of utmost importance to definitely diagnose or exclude EPI. Blood tests do not require cumbersome invasive tests, the taking of large amounts of the patient's time, radiation protection or radiography equipment, or a need for patients to fast overnight. Hence, with sophisticated laboratories possible in-house and worldwide, blood tests can be rapidly applied and the results can be made available typically within hours to days. Four selections of EPI blood tests have some diagnostic characteristics, respective advantages, and disadvantages. This chapter sets out that there are both practical and technical challenges. Practical challenges include the availability of GI unicentric centers, costs, lack of objective viable treatment for EPI, and the general need for both ICUs and the physician GI community to continue to follow up.

Understanding Exocrine Pancreatic Insufficiency (EPI): Diagnosis and Management

1. Introduction to Exocrine Pancreatic Insufficiency (EPI)

The exocrine pancreas is key to digestion, producing up to 1.5 litres of enzymes each day in response to food signals. Each enzyme targets a specific nutrient. Three enzymes – lipase, amylase, and protease – break down fat, starch, and protein. Other enzymes target the carbohydrates, fats, and proteins we eat. Lipase is produced as an inactive enzyme, with the body converting it to active lipase in the proximal intestine. Three glands in the pancreas – known as the acinar cells – provide lipase. Unlike other enzymes, these glands can be destroyed by the bowel's own digestion system as lipase is not converted into active form. Pancreatic lipase needs a special protein called colipase (essential for fat digestion) to form an active complex. However, the colipase produced in the pancreas and released as a more than sufficient amount in direct response to fats but can run out during the process of a heavy meal or in liquid meal excess. Pancreatic colipase becomes essential when caloric intake of a meal exceeds 20 grams of fat or there is an excess of liquid contents in the stomach which dilutes both the pancreatic enzymes.

Exocrine pancreatic insufficiency (EPI) means the pancreas is unable to perform normally. It's the pancreas' role to produce enzymes for food digestion. Without these enzymes, the human body could break down food, allowing nutrients to be absorbed. There are more than 10 different causes of EPI, including cystic fibrosis and chronic pancreatitis. The most common cause is celiac disease. Symptoms can start during childhood. The condition can be difficult to diagnose as the CTRC – a protein which helps diagnose EPI – tends to disappear over time. As many as 4.6% of the UK population may have EPI. EPI is also commonly found in people with irritable bowel syndrome (IBS).

2. Signs and Symptoms of EPI

Affected dogs will often show: greasy or very low firmness in bowel movements; very bad odours in stools; flatulence in some but occasional or no flatulence in others; variable discomfort after eating that is difficult to assess; some dogs may be ravenous if having lost weight. Some dogs may lose weight and have a poor hair coat. Some animals, such as cats, may develop pancreatitis concurrent with EPI and/or IBD. Other symptoms can occur depending on how long EPI has been present (hyperkeratosis, low albumin, fat-soluble vitamin deficiencies, and lipid differences). It is, however, common that mixed canine and feline EPI cases will develop complications of IBD and/or EPI.

In moderate to severe cases of EPI, there are more related identifiable symptoms of malabsorption, poor nutrition, or pain due to underlying disease. These are seen quite rapidly with abrupt losses of normal function over baseline reserves in average or low pancreatic function patients. The extent and duration of pancreatic insufficiency will vary, with effects on digestion and absorption of solid food less than those for fats and carbohydrates. Clinical indications of fat and protein malabsorption usually appear first with carbohydrate malabsorption taking longer to become apparent.

EPI rarely has straightforward or obvious signs or symptoms. This is because the clinical presentation of EPI is highly variable, largely due to the very high reserve in normal pancreatic function and the variety of ways in which absorption of nutrients may be affected. Causes of a mild form of EPI can be wide and varied and often not life-threatening. For many of the causes of mild EPI, if not indicated by related symptoms, treatment may not be necessary.

3. Diagnostic Approaches for EPI

The diagnosis of EPI remains a challenge. Available tests to diagnose EPI are diverse and range from easy to complex, invasive to non-invasive, involving large or small peak activation of pancreatic enzymes, and include several commercial tests. Fecal or plasma/serum assessments for fat or elastase (fat or pancreas markers, respectively), or a functional test are used to diagnose EPI or treatment response to pancreatic enzyme replacement therapy (PERT) in clinical situation. The main purpose of fecal or blood tests to diagnose EPI is to measure excreted or leaked pancreatic enzymes or to measure the consequences of reduced exocrine pancreatic function. The remaining enzymes are expected to be partly destroyed in the gut by the enzyme-unstable environment.

Several approaches are used to diagnose exocrine pancreatic insufficiency (EPI) - phenotyping of maldigestion. Based on Munich consensus reports, pancreatic function tests (PFTs) and fecal fat estimations (FFE) were given a grade I recommendation because they are valid and available. The gold standard for EPI diagnosis is a direct or indirect PFT such as the pancreolauryl test, secretin test, bentiromide test, and 13C-labeled mixed triglyceride breath test. The level of steatorrhea does not correlate with the degree of fat malabsorption because excess fat in diets is absorbed at low enzyme concentrations. Bentiromide requires post-administration urine collection to demonstrate excreted hippuric acid, and

13C-labeled mixed triglycerides collect less than 10% of carbon-13 in feces. Blood tests, such as serum trypsinogen, are widely validated in clinical practice for exams; however, many companies do not offer values above the cut-off at greater than 200 or 250 ng/mL. The most frequent and simple exam used was the coefficient of fat absorption, which detected enzyme deficits of up to 90% accuracy.

3.1. Blood Tests for EPI

Serum trypsin is one of the first enzymes to be created and secreted in the intestine. Since fecal measurement is difficult, direct pancreatic secretion measurement is widely used. Currently there are not so many physicians who measure blood, there are facilities where it can be measured in various forms according to the analyzer installed. One of them is a pancreas-specific amylase (P-TYPEA) that appeals to cardiac surgeons, urologists, and orthopedic surgeons before surgery to explain whether diabetes is caused by pancreatic diabetes or is caused by another. As an additional inspection for patients undergoing gastrectomy, we are testing exocrine function. A blood test for serum trypsin and serum direct bilirubin in patients with chronic pancreatitis has been approved to be tested by public health insurance, and patients are also undergoing these tests. Currently, in addition to the measurement items approved this time, some doctors are conducting additional tests to evaluate the non-returning function by measuring GIP and GLP-1.

Endocrine function of the pancreas is routinely available as noninvasive, indirectly assessing surrogate proteins. These would be to check for serum amylase and lipase. Besides, fasting blood sugar (FBS) and HbA1c are very critical.

Classification of EPI: 3.1 Blood Tests for EPI

3.2. Stool Tests for EPI

The presence of neutral starch in stools is assessed by Lugol's iodine with a specificity of 89-97% and significantly decreased cost compared to a pair of chemistries (sodium rhodizonate with and without α-amylase) selected to account for the different baseline starch content in infants. Combination of the two tests reveals a specificity of 87-100%. For assessments of sugar levels, reading orthotoluidine stability and reducing of sugar colors had a specificity of 49-85% for clinically significant differences that are indiscernible using routine methodology like a Fletcher analyzer for enzymatic measurement of reducing substances.

To measure the caloric content of stools, the van de Kamer test (also known as the O'Sullivan and Maher test) uses an ether solvent to dissolve out the fats from stools. The fats are measured by volume, and 9.3 calories are assumed per milliliter of extracted fat. Since 3 g or 6 g dietary fat is recommended per kilogram per day intake for males and females, respectively, whose weight falls within the normal range for age and height, this standard gives a basis to calculate normal stool fat excretion. In clinical practice, the more rapid, gravimetric, Sudan III stain, or Burkon-Ulz method is the method of choice for 72- to 100-hour stool collections at most facilities and has a specificity of 94-99%.

To increase the sensitivity of the indirect test, quantification of the amount of fat and other nutrients in the stool can be performed. This stool test is often done over a 3-4 day period and is referred to by many names: 72-, 88-, or 100-hour stool study, fecal fat test, or fecal weight test. Stool tests are important in confirming the diagnosis of EPI and also provide baseline measures of fat content in the stool to evaluate the effectiveness of care.

4. Differential Diagnosis of EPI

One of the most challenging aspects of this condition is to differentiate between the various overlapping and frequently coexisting differential diagnoses such as dietary sensitivities, food intolerance, or IBD (especially with small intestinal bacterial overgrowth). Other differentials include exocrine pancreatic dysfunction, lymphangiectasia, colitis, short bowel syndrome, pancreatic and non-pancreatic exocrine dysfunction (due to previous diseases or IBD), other liver diseases, and adrenal insufficiency in the cat. Examining past medication and symptom development can be helpful in narrowing the list of potential diagnoses, as many of the diseases exhibit differential diagnosis may have unique clinical features. Pathobiology might help exclude other causes if performed on feces in case of diarrhea, particularly for food intolerance. Year-round clinical signs are not suggestive of dietary sensitivity. A trial with a hydrolyzed diet for young cats (<6 years old) may be attempted to see whether this will solve the problem: an adverse food reaction may be overgrown by the atypical response to steroids. Dose doses of prednisolone can result in inappetence in cats. Non-responsive EPI cases, in particular where weight loss, type II fatty liver, or exocrine pancreatic atrophy is present on imaging, may be indicative of paradoxical use of steroids in pancreatitis.

- Presenting symptoms - Age and breed of the animal - Availability of specific investigations - Response to treatment - Seasonal acuity and duration of clinical signs

Exocrine pancreatic insufficiency is often misdiagnosed due to overlapping symptoms with the differential diagnoses. Various factors should be considered in the differential diagnosis, including:

5. Management of EPI

Without children and parents gaining an understanding of EPI, they will be frightened and confused when your child is unwell. Parents can help their child understand EPI by providing support and explaining to their child's friends, peers, and teachers. Children soon grow in their ability to be increasingly responsible and independent for the management of EPI in partnership with their parents. Children will require varying levels of involvement based on how long they have had the diagnosis of EPI, ranging from high to extremely low over a period of time. In regard to enzyme treatment for babies with EPI from birth or diagnosed in utero, we always advocate a minimum of a double regular dose of enzymes for each feed. By upping the dose of enzymes this way for babies feeding by NGT/OGT/CCG (nasogastric, oral, or continuous overnight gastrostomy), any bowel contents will be helped in neutralizing the increased acidity and work more effectively. The timing of enzymes for all who have oral feeds is to give the enzymes immediately before the feed, to improve their ability to mix with the food and require less time to work effectively. No child should have their enzymes placed directly into the oral mucosa and gums; this will cause an oral burn, degrading the tissue and attacking the enamel of the teeth.

Management of EPI aims to reduce malabsorption, symptoms, and long-term sequelae such as malnutrition. The mainstay of management is enzyme replacement therapy with regular dietary advice and support from specialist dietitians. Even one-fourth of the normal dose of enzymes can be enough, tailored to the following: age, weight, diet, severity of bowel symptoms, and response to treatment. The overall aim of dietary management is to maintain your child or patient's nutritional status and provide symptom control to allow normal growth and development.

5.1. Enzyme Replacement Therapy

Although low dose and high dose pancrelipase have not been studied directly, high dose pancrelipase has been shown to offer more favorable outcomes for absorption of fat and possibility of improving overall clinical symptoms associated with EPI. Thus, higher doses of PERT are generally recommended. Altered release products are not recommended as they have not been shown to be more effective than immediate release pancrelipase. The measuring unit of enzymes is given in FIP units (Pharmaceutical International Units). Treatment with PERT may help children with EPI to grow and gain weight at a rate expected for their age. The increase in the number and size of stools seen in EPI can be reduced by treatment with PERT (smaller, fewer stools).

Enzyme replacement therapy is the mainstay of treatment for EPI. Pancreatic enzyme replacement therapy, often dosed generally as 25,000 to 40,000 IU of lipase, is used with all ingested meals and snacks. A multicenter, placebo-controlled randomized clinical trial in adult patients with symptoms suggesting EPI, in whom EPI was diagnosed by low coefficients of fat absorption, showed that pancrelipase (administered orally), when compared to placebo, significantly improved steatorrhea by reducing mL/day fat while normalizing the coefficient of fat absorption. This therapy has also been shown to improve abdominal pain, bloating, fecal urgency, hard stools, and number of bowel movements per day versus placebo. The general dose for adults is assessed in units of lipase activity required to control steatorrhea. This enzyme is given with meals and snacks.

5.2. Nutritional Support

As protein and fat digestion, as well as fat-soluble vitamins and calcium absorption, are impacted the most when enzymes are replaced, adopting a more individualized approach in which support is based on patients' dietary fat tolerance might be an efficient strategy. Patients should be screened for conditions that may affect nutritional status and require specific dietary recommendations or nutritional interventions at the time of EPI diagnosis and management. The decision to support patients should be considered as proposed in the ESPEN guideline on clinical nutrition in chronic pancreatitis and should already be applied in daily practice. In patients requiring nutritional assessment, optimal nutritional care is provided within a team setting as recommended in the guidelines for nutritional support in chronic pancreatitis. Gottschalk et al. demonstrated in a systematic review that early dietary and nutritional counseling is conducted in 30% to 100% of patients with CP or EPI, and dieticians and nurses were involved in 45% to 62% of the patients studied, both in curative and supportive care.

Nutritional support: EPI may lead to varying degrees of both digestive and absorptive dysfunction, which may compromise nutritional status if not managed appropriately. Various studies suggest that there is a subpopulation of EPI patients with ongoing malabsorption; however, malnutrition is only observed in a small number of patients. The vast majority of patients with EPI do not develop malnutrition, whereas more patients may experience weight loss or a reduction in median BMI. Nutritional support is of great importance to effectively manage exocrine pancreatic insufficiency.

6. Complications Associated with Untreated EPI

EPI can be associated with and cause a number of complications. Some studies have evaluated the potential complications associated with EPI. In patients with chronic pancreatitis, EPI is associated with osteoporosis and low bone density. EPI was reported in 40% of patients with irritable bowel syndrome with diarrhea and only 15% of patients with irritable bowel syndrome without diarrhea, which was a significant difference. Furthermore, a study of Italian patients found that IBS-D was diagnosed in 18.4% of patients with EPI. Although this did not reach statistical significance, it suggests an important trend and highlights that it may be useful to test for EPI in patients with diarrhea. Management of EPI in patients with IBS: Patients with EPI and IBS-D who underwent diagnostic testing for EPI.

EPI is a common condition of the pancreas that affects the body's ability to break down and absorb nutrients, with some people affected more severely than others. EPI symptoms, if left untreated, can lead to complications including poor growth and cognitive development in children, osteopenia and osteoporosis, anemia, nutrient malabsorption, nutrient deficiency, involuntary weight loss, loss of lean body mass, reduced quality and length of life. With a risk of these complications, accurate diagnosis and management of EPI are important for reducing the risk and impact of these complications.

Exocrine pancreatic insufficiency (EPI) is a condition in which the pancreas does not produce sufficient enzymes to break down and absorb nutrients. If left untreated, the consequences can be significant.

7. Prognosis and Quality of Life in EPI

EPI leads to paucity of pancreatic enzymes so that essential nutrients are incompletely digested, resulting in maldigestion and malabsorption. This can make it difficult for some patients with EPI to manage their disease with medications, leading to potential issues with fat-malabsorption symptoms and also folklore about enzyme harming the patient or how medicines containing animal-derived products are not suitable. The impact of maldigestion depends largely on its severity, efficacy of treatment, as well as other gastrointestinal complications and comorbidities. As such, not all EPI patients would be affected in the same way. Recent patient consultation in EPI post-marketing study shows that the different variation of lifestyles, food culture and dietary habits can affect the different dietary choice even in the different level of EPI severity. Importantly, not only signs of malnutrition can result from EPI and lead to disability, but also problems with bloating, abdominal pain, diarrhea, weight loss and fatigue can lead to a reduction in quality of life. Factors which have been suggested to impact upon wellbeing in affected individuals may include socio-economic status and psychosocial aspects, such as general support, stigma, impact on employment and care provision.

Quality of life (QOL)

The course of EPI is variable and depends most importantly on the underlying disease causing the EPI, and the natural history of that condition. In the case of cystic fibrosis (CF), EPI is one component of the spectrum of disease that is linked to the severity of the genotype. Likelihood of survival for infants born with EPI is high with appropriate EPI treatment. However, in other disorders where EPI is part of their disease, prognosis will vary depending on the disease. Rarer causes of EPI have poor prognosis, usually because of diagnosis occurring late when ill health has generally started causing symptoms. Long-term prognosis can be affected by complications of EPI, such as vitamin deficiencies and impaired fat absorption. The degree of these complications will vary between individuals and is usually related to the severity of their EPI.

Prognosis

8. Research and Future Directions in EPI

However, the future holds many promising directions for EPI research. The development of new technology, such as pancreQuantoTM, describes mesotrypsin quantitation and pancreatic elastase quantitation in a single test, may improve the diagnosis of all stages of pancreatic disease including SAP. Trials showing relatively high sensitivity and specificity are partial verification trials. These trials specifically request that patients with a positive index test undergo the reference standard (blood trypsin concentration). In practice, these patients are usually referred for further investigation because of a high index test result and are therefore more likely to have the target condition of EPI. Such trial designs have been used in EPI but recruitment can be difficult. Future studies of these tests under these conditions are still required in order to define their diagnostic accuracy. Methodological evaluation of diagnostic fraud and diagnostic trials. Current target populations for exocrine pancreatic insufficiency and determination of functional cutoff values for the feline serum.

The main areas of research in EPI include the definition of the disease and the diagnostic tests. Future research will include the development of small animal models that may address some of the underlying factors in EPI. The receiver-operating characteristic (ROC) curve is used to evaluate the accuracy of a test. The area under the ROC curve ranges between 0 and 1. 0.5 indicates the test is worthless, whereas a value of 1 indicates perfect diagnostic accuracy. ROC curves are used to find the optimal cut-off value for a test, i.e. the value with the highest accuracy.

Research and Future Directions